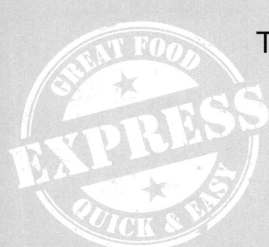

THE *Skinny*
SOUP
RECIPE BOOK

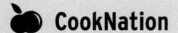

THE SKINNY EXPRESS SOUP RECIPE BOOK
QUICK & EASY, DELICIOUS, LOW CALORIE SOUP RECIPES. ALL UNDER 100, 200, 300 & 400 CALORIES.

ISBN 978-1-909855-95-3

A CIP catalogue record of this book is available from the British Library

Photography: Kongsak/shutterstock

DISCLAIMER

Some recipes may contain nuts or traces of nuts. Those suffering from any allergies associated with nuts should avoid any recipes containing nuts or nut based oils.

This information is provided and sold with the knowledge that the publisher and author do not offer any legal or other professional advice. In the case of a need for any such expertise consult with the appropriate professional.

This book does not contain all information available on the subject, and other sources of recipes are available. This book has not been created to be specific to any individual's requirements.

Every effort has been made to make this book as accurate as possible. However, there may be typographical and or content errors. Therefore, this book should serve only as a general guide and not as the ultimate source of subject information.

This book contains information that might be dated and is intended only to educate and entertain.

The author and publisher shall have no liability or responsibility to any person or entity regarding any loss or damage incurred, or alleged to have incurred, directly or indirectly, by the information contained in this book.

www.cooknationbooks.com
www.bellmackenzie.com

CONTENTS

UNDER 300 CALORIES

INTRODUCTION

Our EXPRESS soups help make losing weight simple, with a no fuss approach and delicious results.

Soup – what could be better? A bowl of warmth that attracts the senses, is full of nutrition, healthy, filling, quick & easy and low in calories. The perfect partner for anyone who is looking to lose weight or maintain a healthy lifestyle.

The Skinny Express Soup Recipe Book creates wonderful soups using tasty fresh ingredients and low calorie alternatives to more traditional soups. Most recipes can be cooked and prepared under 30 minutes using easily obtainable store cupboard and fresh ingredients.

Our EXPRESS soups help make losing weight simple, with a no fuss approach and delicious results. Every bowl falls between 100, 200, 300 or 400 calories: making it easy for you to stick to a calorie controlled plan.

One of the biggest complaints from anyone who is following a diet is the feeling of hunger. Soup really helps, as it is a filling meal in itself. The use of protein, beans, vegetables grains or noodles all in one bowl keeps the hunger pangs away for longer: making it less likely you will want to snack between meals.

One of the most attractive benefits of soup is its versatility. It can come in many forms from a traditional vegetable to broth to an apple & beetroot consommé or Japanese ramen noodle soup. Eating soup opens up a world of healthy, low calorie, low fat alternatives and is the perfect way to clean up your diet while awaking your taste buds to new and sometimes more adventurous alternatives.

EXPRESS – GREAT SOUP IN MINUTES

Many are discouraged from cooking soup at home by the effort of making a rich stock to begin with and sourcing a number of ingredients, which may not form part of the everyday kitchen store cupboard. While a great homemade stock can really be the 'bones' of a good soup, our skinny express recipes offer quicker alternatives without compromising on flavour. For example there are a number of very good quality read made stocks available in every supermarket although we do offer some good simple stock recipes to get you started if you prefer to make yourself. All our recipes fall below either 100, 200, 300 or 400 calories per serving and can be prepared and cooked in around 20 minutes or less. By calculating the number of calories for each dish we've made it easy for you to count your daily calorie intake as part of a controlled diet or a balanced healthy eating plan.

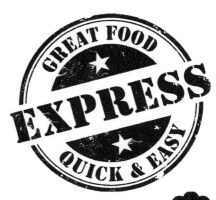

WHAT THIS BOOK WILL DO FOR YOU

The recipes in this book are all low calorie dishes that make it easy for you to control your overall daily calorie intake. The recommended daily calories are 2000 for women and 2500 for men. Broadly speaking, by consuming this level of calories each day you should maintain your current weight. Reducing the number of calories (a calorie deficit) will result in losing weight. This happens because the body begins to use fat stores for energy to make up the reduction in calories, which in turn results in weight loss. Preparing a number of balanced meals throughout the day and counting each calorie however can be difficult, that's why our skinny express soups are so great. We have already counted the calories for each dish making it easy for you to fit this into to your daily eating plan whether you are looking to lose weight, maintain your current figure or are just looking for some great-tasting soup ideas.

I'M ALREADY ON A DIET. CAN I USE THESE RECIPES?

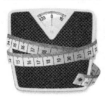

Yes of course. All the recipes can be great accompaniments to many of the popular calorie-counting diets. We all know that sometimes dieting can result in hunger pangs, cravings and boredom from eating the same old foods day in and day out. Skinny express soups can break that cycle by providing filling 'meals in one' that satisfy you for hours afterwards.

I AM ONLY COOKING FOR ONE. WILL THIS BOOK WORK FOR ME?

Yes. To make the best use of each dish we have made all servings for four people. Remember you can always refrigerate or freeze portions for another day if you are just cooking for one.

SOUP IS JUST FOR COLD WINTER NIGHTS, RIGHT?

Wrong! While there is nothing better than a bowl of comforting steaming hot broth on a miserable winter's day, soup isn't just for dark cold nights. It can be a vibrant and refreshing alternative on the brightest and hottest of days , and make use of the best seasonal ingredients all year round. Did you know that some soups can also be served chilled? What could be better on a summer's day? Soups can be a wonderful revelation to your day, waking up your taste buds to new possibilities. Think Thai, Chicken & Coconut or Japanese Ramen Noodle Soup and suddenly you have opened yourself up to a world of soup possibilities.

WHAT MAKES A GREAT SOUP?

Thankfully you don't have to be a great chef to make an incredible soup. There are however a few key elements to making a great soup.

The Base: the start to most soups requires a few vegetables to give your soup a rounded flavour. Onions, carrots and celery are a great start.

Stock: A good quality stock will make the world of difference to the quality of your soup. Use either vegetable, fish or meat stock and if you can make these at home, all the better. You can follow these simple instructions to make homemade stock. If you opt for store-bought stock try to choose a good quality product that is not high in sodium.

Ingredients: Soup is so versatile that almost any ingredient can be used whether you are looking for a meaty protein packed dish, an Asian seafood soup, or a thick vegetarian broth using beans and pulses. Certain ingredients will change the consistency of your soup too, for example potatoes and lentils will thicken, while adding some single cream will make it smoother.

Seasoning: Most soups will require some seasoning. Be careful when choosing your stock that it is not overly high in its sodium content. There are also many popular herbs that compliment soups such as marjoram, thyme, parsley, sage, rosemary, oregano and of course salt and pepper. You should also feel free to experiment. For example: Garlic, ginger and coriander can work well in Asian soups while cumin, turmeric or garam masala can give an authentic Indian feel to your dish.

Garnish: There is nothing better than serving a homemade soup with a little garnish, which not only looks the part but also adds an extra taste. Depending on your dish, freshly chopped herbs, croutons, a little cream, crème fraiche or freshly grated parmesan are all great finishing touches.

ALL RECIPES ARE A GUIDE ONLY

All the recipes in this book are a guide only. You may need to alter quantities and cooking times to suit your own appliances.

ABOUT COOKNATION

CookNation is the leading publisher of innovative and practical recipe books for the modern, health conscious cook.

CookNation titles bring together delicious, easy and practical recipes with their unique approach - easy and delicious, no-nonsense recipes - making cooking for diets and healthy eating fast, simple and fun.

With a range of #1 best-selling titles - from the innovative 'Skinny' calorie-counted series, to the 5:2 Diet Recipes collection - CookNation recipe books prove that 'Diet' can still mean 'Delicious'!

Turn to the end of this book to browse all CookNation's recipe books

www.cooknationbooks.com
www.bellmackenzie.com

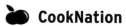 **CookNation**

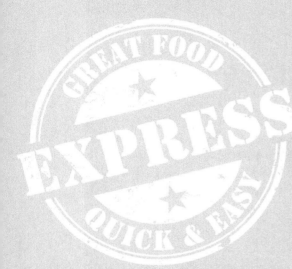

Skinny SOUPS

UNDER 100 CALORIES

SCALLOP TOPPED THAI SOUP

95 calories per serving

Ingredients

- 2 bunches spring onions/scallions, finely chopped
- 2 garlic cloves, crushed
- 3 lemongrass stalks, finely chopped
- 1 tsp each ground coriander/cilantro & ginger
- 1 red chilli, deseeded & finely chopped
- 1lt/4 cups vegetable or chicken stock
- 1 tbsp each Thai fish sauce & brown sugar
- 4 large fresh scallops, cleaned & prepared
- Low cal cooking oil spray
- Salt & pepper to taste

Method

1 Add the all the ingredients, except the scallops, to a large non-stick saucepan. Bring to the boil and gently simmer for 10 minutes.

2 Meanwhile spray the scallops with a little low cal oil and season with salt & pepper. Heat a non-stick frying pan on a medium/high heat and, when the pan is hot, dry fry the scallops for 2-2½ minutes each side or until cooked through.

3 Divide the soup into bowls and serve with a scallop on top.

CHEFS NOTE
Try serving with some lime wedges and freshly chopped coriander.

SIMPLE SAVOY SOUP

98 calories per serving

Ingredients

- 300g/11oz potatoes, peeled & diced
- 1 whole savoy cabbage, shredded
- 1 red chilli, deseeded & finely chopped
- 1.25lt/5 cups vegetable or chicken stock
- Salt & pepper to taste

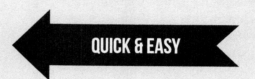

QUICK & EASY

Method

1 Add the all the ingredients to a large non-stick saucepan.

2 Simmer for 10-12 minutes or until the potatoes are tender.

3 Tip the soup into a blender or food processor and whizz until you have a completely smooth texture.

4 Check the seasoning, divide into bowls and serve.

CHEFS NOTE
Serve this simple soup with lots of freshly ground black pepper.

CHILLED CHIVE VICHYSSOISE SOUP

99 calories per serving

Ingredients

- 1 tbsp low fat 'butter' spread
- 1 onion, sliced
- 2 leeks, finely sliced
- 125g/4oz potatoes, peeled & diced
- 750ml/3 cups vegetable or chicken stock
- 250ml/1 cup semi skimmed/half fat milk
- 4 tbsp freshly chopped chives
- Salt & pepper to taste

Method

1 Gently heat the 'butter' in a large non-stick saucepan and add the onion & leeks.

2 Gently sauté for 10-12 minutes until the onions & leek soften. Add the potatoes & stock and simmer for 8-10 minutes or until the potatoes are cooked through.

3 Tip the soup into a blender or food processor and whizz until you have a completely smooth texture.

4 Pass the soup through a sieve, and stir through the milk.

5 Place in a large bowl, cover and leave to cool. When it's cool place in the refrigerator to chill.

6 Serve in shallow bowls with the chopped chives sprinkled over the top.

CHEFS NOTE

Vichyssoise is the classic chilled soup. Add a little low fat cream for a richer finish.

SPINACH & NUTMEG SOUP

95 calories per serving

Ingredients

- 200g/7oz spinach leaves
- 1.25lt/5 cups vegetable or chicken stock
- 120ml/½ cup low fat cream
- ½ tsp each freshly grated nutmeg & ground black pepper
- Salt & pepper to taste

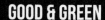

GOOD & GREEN

Method

1 Add the spinach & stock to a large non-stick saucepan, bring to the boil and simmer for a couple of minutes until the spinach is cooked through.

2 Remove from the heat and stir through the cream, nutmeg & pepper.

3 Tip the soup into a blender or food processor and whizz until you have a completely smooth texture.

4 Check the seasoning and serve.

CHEFS NOTE

This is a really quick and easy soup, adjust the nutmeg to suit your own taste.

GAMMON & PEA SOUP

99 calories per serving

Ingredients

- ½ onion, sliced
- 100g/3½oz gammon, finely chopped
- 200g/7oz peas
- 1lt/4 cups vegetable or chicken stock
- Low cal cooking oil spray
- Salt & pepper to taste

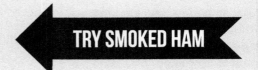
TRY SMOKED HAM

Method

1 Use a little low cal spray to gently sauté the onions & gammon in a large non-stick saucepan, for a few minutes until the onions soften.

2 Add the peas & stock and simmer for 6-8 minutes or until cooked through.

3 Tip the soup into a blender or food processor and whizz until you have a smooth texture.

4 Check the seasoning and serve.

CHEFS NOTE
For a different finish try pulsing the soup rather than blending to a smooth texture.

CLEANSING WATERCRESS & SPINACH SOUP

75 calories per serving

Ingredients

- 2 onions, sliced
- 2 garlic cloves, crushed
- 300g/11oz watercress
- 150g/5oz young spinach leaves
- 1.25lt/5 cups vegetable or chicken stock
- Low cal cooking oil spray
- Salt & pepper to taste

Method

1 Using a little low cal oil gently sauté the onions & garlic in a large non-stick saucepan for a few minutes until the onions soften.

2 Add the watercress, spinach & stock to the pan and simmer for 4 minutes.

3 Tip the soup into a blender or food processor and whizz until you have a completely smooth texture.

4 Check the seasoning and serve.

CHEFS NOTE
Add plenty of black pepper and a swirl of fat free crème fraiche or Greek yogurt when serving if you wish.

ASPARAGUS & CRÈME FRAICHE SOUP

99 calories per serving

Ingredients

- 1 tbsp olive oil
- 1 onion, sliced
- 400g/14oz fresh asparagus
- 1lt/4 cups vegetable or chicken stock
- 4 tbsp fat free crème fraiche
- 2 tbsp freshly chopped flat leaf parsley
- Salt & pepper to taste

Method

1 Gently heat the olive oil in a large non-stick saucepan and sauté the onions for a few minutes until softened.

2 Meanwhile divide the asparagus by cutting off the tips. Put the tips to one side while you chop up the stalks.

3 Add the chopped asparagus stalks to the saucepan and sauté for a further 3 minutes.

4 Add the stock and simmer for 10 minutes or until the chopped asparagus stalks are tender.

5 Tip the soup into a blender or food processor and whizz until you have a completely smooth texture.

6 Return the blended soup to the pan, place on a low heat and add the reserved asparagus tips.

7 Simmer for a few minutes until the tips are tender before stirring through the crème fraiche.

8 Check the seasoning and serve with fresh parsley sprinkled over the top.

CHEFS NOTE
The tip of the asparagus is the flowery end of the stalk.

LIGHT CELERY SOUP

60 calories per serving

Ingredients

- 2 onions, sliced
- 2 garlic cloves, crushed
- 700g/1lb 9oz celery, chopped
- 1.25lt/5 cups vegetable or chicken stock
- Low cal cooking oil spray
- Salt & pepper to taste

Method

1 Gently sauté the onions, garlic & celery in a large non-stick saucepan, with a little low cal spray, for a few minutes until softened.

2 Add the stock and simmer for 8-10 minutes or until the celery is tender.

3 Tip the soup into a blender or food processor and whizz until you have a completely smooth texture.

4 Check the seasoning and serve.

CHEFS NOTE
Try serving with some homemade croutons. Find the recipe on page 82

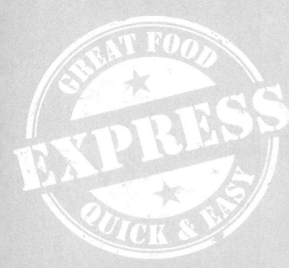

Skinny
SOUPS

UNDER 200 CALORIES

BEETROOT & HORSERADISH SOUP

135 calories per serving

Ingredients

- 1 tbsp olive oil
- 1 onion, sliced
- 600g/1lb 5oz cooked beetroot, chopped
- 1lt/4 cups vegetable or chicken stock
- 4 tbsp fat free Greek yogurt
- 1 tbsp horseradish sauce
- Salt & pepper to taste

Method

1 Gently heat the olive oil in a large non-stick saucepan and sauté the onions for a few minutes until softened.

2 Add the beetroot & stock and simmer for 5-6 minutes or until everything is cooked through and piping hot.

3 Tip the soup into a blender or food processor along with the yogurt & horseradish sauce and whizz until you have a completely smooth texture.

4 Check the seasoning and serve.

CHEFS NOTE
Adjust the quantity of horseradish to suit your own taste.

LIME & PUMPKIN SOUP

165
calories per
serving

Ingredients

- 1 tbsp low fat 'butter' spread
- 1 onion, sliced
- 200g/7oz potatoes, peeled & diced
- 600g/1lb 5oz pumpkin flesh, peeled & diced

- 750ml/3 cups vegetable or chicken stock
- 250ml/1 cup semi skimmed/half fat milk
- 1 lime
- Salt & pepper to taste

Method

1 Heat the 'butter' and gently sauté the onions in a large non-stick saucepan for a few minutes until the onions soften.

2 Add the potatoes, stock & pumpkin and simmer for 10-15 minutes or until everything is tender and piping hot. Stir through the milk and warm for a minute or two before tipping the soup into a blender or food processor.

3 Whizz until you have a completely smooth texture.

4 Cut the lime into wedges and serve each portion of soup with a twist of lime over the top.

CHEFS NOTE
Serve with the lime wedges on the side so that diners can add more lime juice whilst eating.

SQUASH & SPINACH SOUP

180 calories per serving

Ingredients

- 1 onion, sliced
- 2 garlic cloves, crushed
- 400g/14oz potatoes, peeled & diced
- 400g/14oz butternut squash, peeled & diced
- 1lt/4 cups vegetable or chicken stock
- 250g/9oz spinach leaves
- 4 tbsp fat free crème fraiche
- Handful of rocket
- Low cal cooking oil spray
- Salt & pepper to taste

Method

1 Gently sauté the onions, garlic, potatoes & squash in a large non-stick saucepan, with a little low cal spray, for a few minutes until the onions soften (add a splash of water to the pan if you need to loosen it up).

2 Add the stock and simmer for 10-15 minutes or until everything is tender and piping hot. Add the spinach and cook for 2-3 minutes or until fully wilted.

3 Tip the soup into a blender or food processor and whizz until you have a completely smooth texture.

4 Check the seasoning, place a spoonful of crème fraiche into each bowl with a few sprigs of rocket and serve.

CHEFS NOTE

Stir the crème fraiche though the soup or leave as a mound depending on your preference.

BEAN & YOGURT SOUP

180 calories per serving

Ingredients

- 1 onion, sliced
- 2 sticks of celery
- 2 garlic cloves, crushed
- ½ tsp dried thyme
- 1lt/4 cups vegetable or chicken stock
- 50g/2oz rice

- 500g/1lb 2oz broad beans
- 4 tbsp fat free Greek yogurt
- ½ tsp paprika
- Low cal cooking oil spray
- Salt & pepper to taste

Method

1 Using a little low cal spray gently sauté the onions, celery, garlic & thyme in a large non-stick saucepan for a few minutes until softened.

2 Add the stock & rice and simmer for 10 minutes. Add the broad beans and continue to cook until the rice is tender.

3 Tip the soup into a blender or food processor and whizz until you have a completely smooth texture.

4 Check the seasoning and serve with a tablespoon of Greek yogurt swirled though the soup, sprinkle with paprika and serve.

CHEFS NOTE

Unless you are using very tender broad beans you will need to pod them (blanche and skin them).

SUNSHINE PEPPER SOUP

115
calories per
serving

Ingredients

- 1 tbsp olive oil
- 2 onions, sliced
- 2 red peppers, deseeded & sliced
- 2 tbsp mild curry powder
- 1lt/4 cups vegetable or chicken stock

- 300g/11oz tinned pineapple, finely chopped
- 2 tbsp fat free crème fraiche
- Salt & pepper to taste

Method

1 Heat the oil in a large non-stick saucepan and gently sauté the onions & peppers for a few minutes until softened.

2 Stir through the curry powder for a minute or two before adding the stock and pineapple. Simmer for 8-10 minutes or until everything is cooked through and piping hot.

3 Remove from the heat, stir through the crème fraiche until well combined. Check the seasoning and serve.

CHEFS NOTE
This unusual soup makes a fruity change to a soup-day snack.

CHICKEN BROTH

170
calories per serving

Ingredients

- 2 onions, sliced
- 3 celery stalks, chopped
- 200g/7oz carrots, peeled & chopped
- 3 garlic cloves, crushed
- 2 bay leaves
- 1 tbsp white peppercorns

- 2 tbsp freshly chopped flat leaf parsley
- 300g/11oz chicken breast (leave the breast whole)
- 1.25lt/5 cups vegetable or chicken stock
- Salt & pepper to taste

Method

1 Add all the ingredients to a large non-stick saucepan, bring to the boil and simmer for 15-20 minutes or until the chicken is cooked through.

2 Remove the chicken breast and put to one side.

3 Meanwhile pass the soup through a sieve to create a clear broth. Return the soup to the pan and place on a gentle heat.

4 Use two forks to shred the chicken breast. Add the shredded chicken back to the pan and warm through for a few minutes.

5 Check the seasoning and serve.

CHEFS NOTE
This is a simple clear broth. Perfect for a light lunch on wintry days.

BEAN & LENTIL SOUP WITH MUSTARD CREAM

170 calories per serving

Ingredients

- 1 onion, sliced
- 2 garlic cloves, crushed
- 2 stalks of celery, chopped
- 200g/7oz carrots, peeled & chopped
- 200g/7oz tinned white beans, drained and rinsed
- 2 ripe tomatoes, chopped
- 50g/2oz puy lentils
- 1lt/4 cups vegetable or chicken stock
- 4 tbsp fat free crème fraiche
- 1 tbsp Dijon mustard
- 1 tbsp finely chopped flat leaf parsley
- Low cal cooking oil spray
- Salt & pepper to taste

Method

1 Using a little low cal spray, gently sauté the onions, garlic, celery & carrots in a large non-stick saucepan for a few minutes until softened (add a splash of water to loosen it up if needed).

2 Add the beans, tomatoes, lentils & stock and simmer for 12-16 minutes or until the lentils are tender.

3 Tip the soup into a blender or food processor and whizz until you have a completely smooth texture.

4 Mix together the crème fraiche, mustard and parsley and swirl through each bowl of soup.

CHEFS NOTE

Alter the quantity of mustard to suit your own taste.

CARROT & DOUBLE CORIANDER SOUP

105 calories per serving

Ingredients

- 1 onion, sliced
- 2 garlic cloves, crushed
- 600g/1lb 5oz carrots, peeled & chopped
- 1 tsp ground coriander/cilantro
- 1lt/4 cups vegetable or chicken stock
- 4 tbsp fat free Greek yogurt
- 4 tbsp freshly chopped coriander/cilantro
- Low cal cooking oil spray
- Salt & pepper to taste

Method

1 Using a little low cal spray gently sauté the onions & garlic in a large non-stick saucepan for a few minutes until softened (add a splash of water to loosen it up if needed).

2 Add the carrots, ground coriander & stock and simmer for 8-12 minutes or until the carrots are tender.

3 Tip the soup into a blender or food processor and whizz until you have a completely smooth texture.

4 Check the seasoning, swirl a tablespoon of yogurt through each bowl of soup and sprinkle with freshly chopped coriander.

CHEFS NOTE
Add a little more stock to alter the consistency of the soup if you wish.

TOMATO & BASIL CROUTON SOUP

150 calories per serving

Ingredients

- 4 portions homemade croutons (see page 82 for recipe)
- 1 tbsp olive oil
- 1 red onion, finely chopped
- 4 garlic cloves, crushed
- 1 tbsp tomato puree

- ½ tsp crushed sea salt
- 800g/1¾lb tinned chopped tomatoes
- 250ml/1 cup vegetable or chicken stock
- 4 tbsp freshly chopped basil
- Salt & pepper to taste

Method

1 Gently heat the olive oil in a large non-stick saucepan and add the chopped onions & garlic. Sauté for a few minutes until the onions soften.

2 Stir through the puree, add the salt, chopped tomatoes, stock & basil and simmer for 10-12 minutes or until everything is cooked though and piping hot.

3 Sprinkle in the croutons, check the seasoning and serve.

CHEFS NOTE
Try making your own croutons using the recipe on page 82.

CREAMY BROCCOLI & STILTON SOUP

175 calories per serving

Ingredients

- 1 tbsp olive oil
- 4 shallots, chopped
- 1 garlic clove, crushed
- 50g/2oz rice
- 500g/1lb 2oz broccoli florets
- 1lt/4 cups vegetable or chicken stock
- 2 tbsp fat free crème fraiche
- 50g/2oz low fat Stilton cheese
- Salt & pepper to taste

Method

1 Gently heat the olive oil in a large non-stick saucepan and add the shallots & garlic.

2 Sauté for a few minutes until the shallots soften.

3 Add the rice, broccoli florets & stock and simmer for 12-16 minutes or until the rice is tender.

4 Tip the soup into a blender or food processor, along with the crème fraiche, and whizz until you have a completely smooth texture.

5 Check the seasoning and serve with the Stilton cheese crumbled over the top.

CHEFS NOTE
Use mild onions if you don't have shallots to hand.

PARSLEY & POTATO SOUP

150 calories per serving

Ingredients

- 1 tbsp low fat 'butter' spread
- 1 onion, sliced
- 2 garlic cloves, crushed
- 1 tsp crushed sea salt
- 200g/7oz mushrooms, finely chopped
- 400g/14oz potatoes, peeled & diced
- Large bunch flat leaf parsley
- 1lt/4 cups vegetable or chicken stock
- 250ml/1 cup semi skimmed/half fat milk
- 2 tbsp freshly chopped flat leaf parsley
- Salt & pepper to taste

Method

1 Gently heat the 'butter' in a large non-stick saucepan and add the onions, garlic, salt, mushrooms & diced potatoes.

2 Sauté for a few minutes, cover and leave on a very low heat to 'sweat' for about 6 minutes.

3 Add the parsley & stock and simmer for 8-10 minutes or until the potatoes are tender.

4 Tip the soup into a blender or food processor and whizz until you have a completely smooth texture.

5 Return the blended soup to the pan, place on a low heat and stir through the milk until well combined.

6 Check the seasoning and serve.

CHEFS NOTE

This soup is a lovely vibrant colour. Serve with plenty of black pepper.

GREEK BEETROOT SOUP

SERVES 4

155 calories per serving

Ingredients

- 1 tbsp olive oil
- 1 onion, sliced
- 1 garlic clove, crushed
- 600g/1lb 5oz cooked beetroot, chopped
- 1.25lt/5 cups vegetable or chicken stock
- 75g/3oz low fat Greek feta cheese
- Salt & pepper to taste

Method

1 Gently heat the olive oil in a large non-stick saucepan and sauté the onions and garlic for a few minutes until softened.

2 Add the beetroot & stock and simmer for 5-6 minutes or until everything is cooked through and piping hot.

3 Tip the soup into a blender or food processor and whizz until you have a completely smooth texture.

4 Check the seasoning and serve in shallow bowls with the feta cheese crumbled over the top.

CHEFS NOTE

Make sure you use low fat feta cheese to keep your soup 'skinny'.

BLENDED BROCCOLI & CAPER SOUP

160 calories per serving

Ingredients

- 1 tbsp olive oil
- 1 onion, sliced
- 1 garlic clove, crushed
- 200g/7oz fresh tomatoes, chopped
- 600g/1lb 5oz broccoli florets, chopped

- 6 tbsp capers, drained & rinsed
- 1lt/4 cups vegetable or chicken stock
- 2 tbsp fat free Greek yogurt
- Salt & pepper to taste

Method

1 Gently heat the olive oil in a large non-stick saucepan and add the onion, garlic & tomatoes.

2 Sauté for a few minutes before adding the broccoli florets, capers & stock. Simmer for 6-8 minutes or until the broccoli is tender.

3 Tip the soup into a blender or food processor and whizz until you have a completely smooth texture.

4 Check the seasoning and serve with a dollop of yogurt in the centre.

CHEFS NOTE
Try using young tenderstem broccoli if it is in season.

MARIS PIPER SOUP

190 calories per serving

Ingredients

- 1 tbsp low fat 'butter' spread
- 1 onion, sliced
- 1 tsp crushed sea salt
- 600g/1lb 5oz Maris Piper potatoes, peeled & diced
- 1lt/4 cups vegetable or chicken stock
- 250ml/1 cup semi skimmed/half fat milk
- 2 tbsp freshly chopped flat leaf parsley
- Salt & pepper to taste

Method

1 Gently heat the 'butter' in a large non-stick saucepan and add the onions, salt & diced potatoes.

2 Sauté for a few minutes, cover and leave on a very low heat to 'sweat' for about 8 minutes.

3 Add the stock and simmer for 8-10 minutes or until the potatoes are tender.

4 Tip the soup into a blender or food processor and whizz until you have a completely smooth texture.

5 Return the blended soup to the pan, place on a low heat and stir through the milk until well combined.

6 Check the seasoning and serve with fresh parsley sprinkled over the top.

CHEFS NOTE
Maris Piper potatoes are particularly good for simple soup but any kind of white floury potato will work well.

DOUBLE ONION SOUP

120 calories per serving

Ingredients

- 1 tbsp olive oil
- 2 red onions, peeled & sliced
- 2 white onions, peeled & sliced
- 1 tbsp brown sugar
- 1 tbsp plain/all purpose flour
- 1.25lt/5 cups vegetable or chicken stock
- Salt & pepper to taste

Method

1 Heat the olive oil in a large non-stick saucepan and gently sauté the onions for a few minutes until softened.

2 Add the brown sugar and stir through until dissolved.

3 Stir through the flour and cook for a further 2 minutes before adding the stock (add the stock a little at a time and stir continuously).

4 Bring to the boil and cook for 10 minutes.

5 Check the seasoning and serve.

CHEFS NOTE

Red onions will give this soup a stronger taste, substitute for mild onions if you prefer.

COCONUT CREAM & LIME SOUP

195
calories per serving

Ingredients

- 1 onion, sliced
- 1 garlic clove, crushed
- 1 tsp freshly grated ginger
- 800g/1¾lb sweet potatoes, peeled & diced
- 1lt/4 cups vegetable or chicken stock
- 2 tbsp coconut cream
- Zest of 1 lime
- Low cal cooking oil spray
- Salt & pepper to taste

Method

1 Using a little low cal spray gently sauté the onions, garlic & ginger in a large non-stick saucepan, for a few minutes until the onions soften (add a splash of water to the pan if you need to loosen it up).

2 Add the sweet potatoes & stock and simmer for 15-20 minutes or until the sweet potatoes are cooked through.

3 Add the coconut cream and tip the soup into a blender or food processor. Whizz until you have a completely smooth texture.

4 Check the seasoning and serve in shallow bowls with the lime zest sprinkled over the top.

CHEFS NOTE

Lime wedges served on the side are also good to 'lift' the soup a little when eating.

CLASSIC TOMATO SOUP

155
calories per
serving

Ingredients

- 1 tbsp olive oil
- 1 onion, sliced
- 2 garlic cloves, crushed
- 250g/9oz carrots
- 800g/1¾lb ripe tomatoes

- 1 tsp brown sugar
- 250ml/1 cup tomato passata/sieved tomatoes
- 1lt/4 cups vegetable or chicken stock
- Salt & pepper to taste

Method

1 Gently heat the olive oil in a large non-stick saucepan and sauté the onions and garlic for a few minutes until softened.

2 Add the carrots, tomatoes & sugar and cook for a further 3-4 minutes until the sugar dissolves.

3 Add the tomato passata & stock and simmer for 8-10 minutes or until the carrots are tender.

4 Tip the soup into a blender or food processor and whizz until you have a completely smooth texture.

5 Check the seasoning and serve.

CHEFS NOTE
Fresh chopped herbs and/or a swirl of low fat cream are a great addition to this simple soup.

APPLE & CAULIFLOWER SOUP

175 calories per serving

Ingredients

- 1 tbsp olive oil
- 1 onion, sliced
- 800g/1¾lb cauliflower florets
- 1lt/4 cups vegetable or chicken stock
- 2 eating apples, peeled, cored & chopped
- 250ml/1 cup semi skimmed/half fat milk
- Salt & pepper to taste

Method

1 Gently heat the olive oil in a large non-stick saucepan and sauté the onions for a few minutes until softened.

2 Add the cauliflower florets, stock & apples and simmer for 8-10 minutes or until the cauliflower is tender.

3 Tip the soup into a blender or food processor and whizz until you have a completely smooth texture.

4 Return the blended soup to the pan, place on a low heat and stir through the milk until well combined.

5 Check the seasoning and serve.

CHEFS NOTE
Use sweet eating apples rather than cooking apples for this subtle soup.

SPICED SMOOTH CARROT SOUP

145 calories per serving

Ingredients

- 1 tbsp olive oil
- 1 onion, sliced
- 2 garlic cloves, crushed
- ½ tsp each ground cumin, turmeric & coriander/cilantro
- 200g/7oz potatoes, peeled & chopped
- 800g/1¾lb carrots, peeled & chopped
- 1lt/4 cups vegetable or chicken stock
- Salt & pepper to taste

Method

1 Gently heat the olive oil in a large non-stick saucepan and sauté the onions and garlic for a few minutes until softened.

2 Stir through the dried spices and add the potatoes, carrots & stock. Cover and cook for 10-12 minutes or until the carrots and potatoes are tender.

3 Tip the soup into a blender or food processor and whizz until you have a completely smooth texture.

4 Check the seasoning and serve.

CHEFS NOTE
Add a little more stock if you want to alter the consistency of the soup.

WARMING PUMPKIN SOUP

190
calories per
serving

Ingredients

- 800g/1¾lb pumpkin flesh, cubed
- 1 onion, sliced
- 1 garlic clove, crushed
- 1lt/4 cups vegetable or chicken stock
- ½ tsp each dried thyme & crushed chilli flakes
- 250ml/1 cup low fat coconut milk
- Salt & pepper to taste

Method

1 Put the pumpkin, onion, garlic, stock, thyme & chilli flakes into a saucepan. Bring to the boil and simmer for 10-12 minutes or until the pumpkin flesh is tender.

2 Tip the soup into a blender or food processor and whizz until you have a completely smooth texture.

3 Return the blended soup to the pan, place on a low heat and stir through the coconut milk until well combined.

4 Check the seasoning and serve.

CHEFS NOTE
For extra spice try serving with slivers of finely chopped red chilli sprinkled over the top of the soup.

LEEK & POTATO SOUP

140
calories per
serving

Ingredients

- 4 leeks, sliced
- 2 garlic cloves, crushed
- 400g/14oz potatoes, peeled & diced
- 1 tsp dried thyme
- 1lt/4 cups vegetable or chicken stock

- 250ml/1 cup semi skimmed/half fat milk
- 4 spring onions/scallions, finely sliced lengthways
- Salt & pepper to taste

Method

1 Using a little low cal spray gently sauté the leeks & garlic in a large non-stick saucepan for a few minutes until the leeks soften.

2 Add the potatoes & thyme and sauté for a minute or two longer (add a splash of water to the pan if you need to loosen it up).

3 Add the stock and simmer for 10-15 minutes or until everything is tender and piping hot.

4 Tip the soup into a blender or food processor and whizz until you have a completely smooth texture.

5 Return the soup to the pan and stir through the milk on a gentle heat.

6 Check the seasoning and serve in shallow bowls with the spring onions sprinkled over the top.

CHEFS NOTE
Slice the spring onions in half lengthways. Then slice each half lengthways again into thirds to create thin ribbons.

THYME & CANNELLINI SOUP

199 calories per serving

Ingredients

- 1 onion, sliced
- 2 garlic cloves, crushed
- 75g/3oz lean, back bacon, finely chopped
- 1 tbsp freshly chopped thyme
- 1.25lt/5 cups vegetable or chicken stock
- 600g/1lb 5oz tinned cannellini beans, drained & rinsed
- Low cal cooking oil spray
- Salt & pepper to taste

Method

1 Gently sauté the onion, garlic, bacon & fresh thyme in a large non-stick saucepan, with a little low cal spray, for a few minutes until the onions soften and the bacon is cooked.

2 Add the stock & beans and simmer for 8-10 minutes or until everything is tender and piping hot.

3 Tip the soup into a blender or food processor and whizz until you have a completely smooth texture.

4 Check the seasoning and serve.

CHEFS NOTE
Use dried thyme if you don't have fresh thyme to hand.

BROCCOLI & BLACK PEPPER SOUP

145 calories per serving

Ingredients

- 1 tbsp olive oil
- 1 onion, sliced
- 1 garlic clove, crushed
- 200g/7oz potatoes, peeled & diced
- 500g/21lb 2oz broccoli florets
- 1.25lt/5 cups vegetable or chicken stock
- ½-1 tsp freshly ground black pepper
- Salt & pepper to taste

Method

1 Gently heat the olive oil in a large non-stick saucepan and add the onions, garlic and potatoes. Sauté for a few minutes until the onions soften.

2 Add the broccoli florets & stock and simmer for 8-10 minutes or until the potatoes and broccoli are tender.

3 Tip the soup into a blender or food processor and whizz until you have a completely smooth texture.

4 Serve in shallow bowls with the ground black pepper sprinkled over the top.

CHEFS NOTE
A dollop of fat free Greek yogurt makes a great garnish to this soup.

MEXICAN SPICED SOUP

175 calories per serving

Ingredients

- 1 tbsp olive oil
- 1 onion, sliced
- 2 garlic cloves, crushed
- 1 red pepper, deseeded & sliced
- 400g/14oz tinned kidney beans, rinsed

- 1 tsp each ground cumin & paprika
- ½ tsp chilli powder
- 400g/14oz tinned chopped tomatoes
- 1lt/4 cups vegetable or chicken stock
- Salt & pepper to taste

Method

1 Heat the olive oil in a large non-stick saucepan and gently sauté the onions, garlic and sliced peppers for a few minutes until softened.

2 Add the kidney beans, ground spices, chopped tomatoes & stock and simmer for 8-10 minutes or until everything is tender & piping hot.

3 Place half the soup into a blender or food processor and whizz until you have a completely smooth texture.

4 Return the blended soup to the pan and combine well with the remaining chunky soup.

5 Check the seasoning and serve.

CHEFS NOTE
Try serving with some freshly chopped coriander sprinkled over the top.

MUSHROOM & LEEK SOUP

125
calories per serving

Ingredients

- 1 tbsp olive oil
- 2 leeks, finely sliced
- 2 garlic cloves, crushed
- 300g/11oz chestnut mushrooms, finely chopped

- 2 tbsp plain/all purpose flour
- 750ml/3 cups vegetable or chicken stock
- 250ml/1 cup semi skimmed/half fat milk
- Salt & pepper to taste

Method

1 Heat the olive oil in a large non-stick saucepan and gently sauté the leeks & garlic for a few minutes until softened.

2 Add the mushrooms and cook for 4 minutes. Stir through the flour and cook for a further 2 minutes before adding the stock (add the stock a little at a time and stir continuously).

3 Leave to simmer for 5 minutes. Stir though the milk, check the seasoning and serve.

CHEFS NOTE
Save time on chopping by whizzing the mushrooms in a food processor first.

FENNEL & DILL SOUP

170 calories per serving

Ingredients

- 1 tbsp olive oil
- 1 onion, sliced
- 400g/14oz potatoes, peeled & diced
- 2 fennel bulbs, chopped
- 1lt/4 cups vegetable or chicken stock
- 4 tbsp freshly chopped dill
- Salt & pepper to taste

Method

1 Gently heat the olive oil in a large non-stick saucepan and add the onions. Sauté for a few minutes until softened and then add the potatoes & fennel. Continue to sauté for a few minutes.

2 Add the stock and simmer for 8-10 minutes or until the potatoes are tender.

3 Tip the soup into a blender or food processor with half of the dill and whizz until you have a completely smooth texture.

4 Check the seasoning and serve with the remaining dill sprinkled over the top.

CHEFS NOTE
Add a little milk for a creamier finish.

EASY SWEETCORN & TOMATO SOUP

190 calories per serving

Ingredients

- 1 tbsp olive oil
- 1 onion, sliced
- 2 garlic cloves, crushed
- 1 red pepper, deseeded & sliced
- 1 tsp each ground cumin & paprika

- 400g/14oz frozen sweetcorn
- 800g/1¾lb tinned chopped tomatoes
- 750ml/3 cups vegetable or chicken stock
- Salt & pepper to taste

Method

1 Heat the olive oil in a large non-stick saucepan and gently sauté the onions, garlic and sliced peppers for a few minutes until softened.

2 Add the ground spices, sweetcorn, chopped tomatoes & stock and simmer for 10-15 minutes or until everything is tender & piping hot.

3 Place half the soup into a blender or food processor and whizz until you have a completely smooth texture.

4 Return the blended soup to the pan and combine well with the remaining unblended soup.

5 Check the seasoning and serve.

CHEFS NOTE

This is a super easy store-cupboard soup. Don't bother sautéing the onions if you are short of time. Just add everything to the saucepan and cook.

BACON & BORLOTTI SOUP

180
calories per
serving

Ingredients

- 1 onion, sliced
- 2 garlic cloves, crushed
- 75g/3oz lean, back bacon, finely chopped
- 2 tbsp tomato puree/paste
- 1.25lt/5 cups vegetable or chicken stock
- 500g/1lb 2oz tinned borlotti beans, drained & rinsed
- Low cal cooking oil spray
- Salt & pepper to taste

Method

1 Gently sauté the onion, garlic & bacon in a large non-stick saucepan, with a little low cal spray, for a few minutes until the onions soften and the bacon is cooked.

2 Stir through the tomato puree, add the stock & beans and simmer for 8 minutes.

3 Use the back of a large spoon or fork to crush some of the beans against the side of the pan. Combine well and cook for a further 5 minutes or until everything is piping hot.

4 Check the seasoning and serve.

CHEFS NOTE
Crushing some of the beans will give the soup a chunky base, or you could blend a couple of ladles full and return to the pan for a smoother base.

CHILLED SUMMER SOUP

175
calories per serving

Ingredients

- 1 tbsp olive oil
- 1 onion, sliced
- 2 garlic cloves, crushed
- 800g/1¾lb peas

- 1 iceberg lettuce, roughly chopped
- 1.25lt/5 cups vegetable or chicken stock
- 2 tbsp freshly chopped mint
- Salt & pepper to taste

Method

1 Gently heat the olive oil in a large non-stick saucepan and add the onions & garlic.

2 Sauté for a few minutes until the onions soften.

3 Add the peas, lettuce, stock & mint and simmer for 3-5 minutes or until the peas are cooked through and everything is piping hot.

4 Tip the soup into a blender or food processor and whizz until you have a completely smooth texture.

5 Place in a large bowl, cover and leave to cool. When it's cool place in the refrigerator to chill.

6 Serve in shallow bowls with plenty of black pepper.

CHEFS NOTE
A swirl of low fat cream or crème fraiche, just before serving makes a good addition to this refreshing chilled soup.

CREAMY CAULIFLOWER SOUP

140 calories per serving

Ingredients

- 1 tbsp olive oil
- 1 onion, sliced
- 1 garlic clove, crushed
- 1 tsp each ground coriander/cilantro
- 900g/2lb cauliflower florets
- 1lt/4 cups vegetable or chicken stock
- 250ml/1 cup semi skimmed/half fat milk
- 2 tbsp freshly chopped flat leaf parsley
- Salt & pepper to taste

Method

1 Gently heat the olive oil in a large non-stick saucepan and add the onions and garlic.

2 Sauté for a few minutes until the onions soften and then stir through the ground coriander.

3 Add the cauliflower florets & stock and simmer for 8-10 minutes or until the cauliflower is tender.

4 Tip the soup into a blender or food processor and whizz until you have a completely smooth texture.

5 Return the blended soup to the pan, place on a low heat and stir through the milk until well combined.

6 Check the seasoning and serve with fresh parsley sprinkled over the top.

CHEFS NOTE

For a different taste try substituting half a teaspoon of ground nutmeg in place of the coriander.

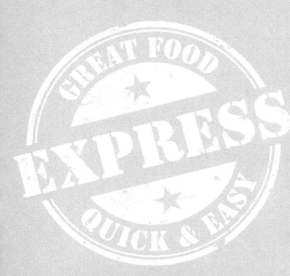

Skinny *SOUPS*

....

UNDER 300 CALORIES

....

CHICKEN & HAM SOUP

215 calories per serving

Ingredients

- 2 onions, sliced
- 200g/7oz carrots, peeled & chopped
- 200g/7oz turnip, peeled & chopped
- 200g/7oz potatoes, peeled & chopped
- 1lt/4 cups vegetable or chicken stock
- 75g/3oz smoked ham, shredded
- 200g/7oz cooked chicken, shredded
- Low cal cooking oil spray
- Salt & pepper to taste

Method

1 Use a little low cal spray to gently sauté the onions in a large non-stick saucepan, for a few minutes until the onions soften.

2 Add the vegetables & stock and simmer for 10-12 minutes or until cooked through.

3 Tip the soup into a blender or food processor and whizz until you have a smooth texture.

4 Return to the pan and add the shredded ham & chicken. Warm through, check the seasoning and serve.

CHEFS NOTE
Add a little more stock if you want to alter the consistency of the soup.

SUPERFAST SPICY MISO SOUP

225 calories per serving

Ingredients

- 2 garlic cloves, crushed
- 2 red chillies, deseeded & finely chopped
- ½ tsp ground ginger
- 4 tbsp miso paste

- 1.25lt/5 cups boiling water
- 1 pak choi/bok choi, shredded
- 200g/7oz thin egg noodles
- Salt & pepper to taste

Method

1 Add the water and miso paste to a non-stick saucepan and stir well on a medium heat.

2 Add all the ingredients to the pan and cook for 3-4 minutes or until everything is cooked through and piping hot.

3 Check the seasoning, spoon into bowls and serve.

CHEFS NOTE

Quick and easy, you can add almost any vegetables or shredded meat you like.

BASIL PESTO & SWEET POTATO SOUP

215 calories per serving

Ingredients

- Large bunch of fresh basil
- 2 tbsp olive oil
- ½ tsp crushed sea salt flakes
- 1 onion, chopped
- 3 garlic cloves, crushed
- 800g/1¾lb sweet potatoes, peeled & diced
- 1lt/4 cups vegetable or chicken stock
- Low cal cooking oil spray
- Salt & pepper to taste

Method

1 First make the pesto by finely chopping the basil and combining with the oil & salt. Mix well and set to one side.

2 Using a little low cal spray gently sauté the onions, garlic & sweet potatoes in a large non-stick saucepan for a few minutes until the onions soften (add a splash of water to the pan if you need to loosen it up).

3 Add the stock and simmer for 10-15 minutes or until the sweet potatoes are cooked through.

4 Tip the soup into a blender or food processor and whizz until you have a completely smooth texture.

5 Check the seasoning, pour into bowls and divide the pesto into the centre of each soup bowl.

CHEFS NOTE
The oil in the pesto is used sparingly. Add a little more if you feel the pesto needs it.

EDAMAME & DRESSED YOGURT SOUP

290 calories per serving

Ingredients

- 4 tbsp fat free Greek yogurt
- Large bunch of fresh chopped coriander/cilantro
- 2 onions, chopped
- 1 tsp dried thyme

- 800g/1¾lb podded edamame peas
- 750ml/3 cups vegetable or chicken stock
- 250ml/1 cup semi skimmed/half fat milk
- Low cal cooking oil spray
- Salt & pepper to taste

Method

1 First prepare the yogurt dressing by finely chopping the coriander and combining with the yogurt along with a little salt & pepper. Set to one side while you make the soup.

2 Using a little low cal spray gently sauté the onions in a large non-stick saucepan for a few minutes until the onions soften (add a splash of water to the pan if you need to loosen it up).

3 Add the thyme, peas & stock and simmer for 10-12 minutes or until the peas are cooked through and tender.

4 Tip the soup into a blender or food processor and whizz until you have a completely smooth texture.

5 Return the soup to the pan on a gentle heat and stir through the milk until warmed through.

6 Check the seasoning, pour into bowls and divide the coriander yogurt into the centre of each soup bowl.

CHEFS NOTE

Use seasonal Spring peas or tinned soya beans if you can't source fresh edamame.

CREAMED SWEETCORN SOUP

250 calories per serving

Ingredients

- 2 tbsp olive oil
- 1 onion, sliced
- 2 garlic cloves, crushed
- 300g/11oz potatoes, peeled & chopped
- 400g/14oz sweetcorn
- 1lt/4 cups vegetable or chicken stock
- 3 tbsp fat free crème fraiche
- 2 tbsp freshly chopped chives
- Salt & pepper to taste

Method

1 Gently heat the olive oil in a large non-stick saucepan and sauté the onions & garlic for a few minutes until softened.

2 Add the chopped potatoes, sweetcorn & stock to the saucepan and simmer for 12-14 minutes or until the potatoes are tender.

3 Tip the soup into a blender or food processor along with the crème fraiche and pulse a few times to cream the sweetcorn (but not completely puree it).

4 Check the seasoning and serve with fresh chives sprinkled over the top.

CHEFS NOTE
You could reserve some of the sweetcorn to serve as a garnish along with the chives.

THAI NOODLE SOUP

290
calories per serving

Ingredients

- 2 bunches spring onions/scallions, finely chopped
- 2 garlic cloves, crushed
- 2 lemongrass stalks, finely chopped
- 1 tsp each ground coriander/cilantro & turmeric
- 200g/7oz peeled prawns, roughly chopped
- 1 red chilli, deseeded & finely chopped
- 750ml/3 cups vegetable or chicken stock
- 250ml/1 cup low fat coconut milk
- 1 tbsp Thai fish sauce
- 200g/7oz thin egg noodles
- Salt & pepper to taste

Method

1 Add all the ingredients, except the noodles, to a large non-stick saucepan.

2 Simmer for 6 minutes before adding the noodles.

3 Cook for a couple of minutes longer until the noodles are tender and the prawns are cooked through.

4 Check the seasoning, spoon into bowls and serve.

CHEFS NOTE
Serve with some freshly chopped chilli & coriander.

LEMONGRASS NOODLE SOUP

235 calories per serving

Ingredients

- 2 bunches spring onions/scallions, finely chopped
- 2 garlic cloves, crushed
- 2 lemongrass stalks, finely chopped
- 125g/4oz carrots, sliced into matchsticks
- 1 red chilli, deseeded & finely chopped

- ½ tsp ground ginger
- 1.25lt/5 cups vegetable or chicken stock
- 125g/4oz baby sweetcorn, chopped
- 200g/7oz thin egg noodles
- Salt & pepper to taste

Method

1 Add the all the ingredients, except the noodles, to a large non-stick saucepan.

2 Simmer for 8 minutes before adding the noodles.

3 Cook for a couple of minutes longer until the noodles & carrots are tender.

4 Check the seasoning, spoon into bowls and serve.

CHEFS NOTE
Try serving with some freshly chopped coriander or dill.

MISO CHICKEN NOODLE SOUP

295 calories per serving

Ingredients

- 4 garlic cloves, crushed
- 1 red chilli, deseeded & finely chopped
- ½ tsp ground ginger
- 3 tbsp miso paste
- 1.5lt/6 cups boiling water
- 150g/5oz chicken breast, thinly sliced
- 125g/4oz baby sweetcorn, chopped
- 1 pak choi/bok choi, shredded
- 200g/7oz thin egg noodles
- 75g/3oz sugar snap peas
- Lime wedges to serve
- Low cal cooking oil spray
- Salt & pepper to taste

Method

1 Using a little low cal spray, gently sauté the garlic, red chilli & ginger in a large non-stick saucepan for a few minutes until softened (add a splash of water to loosen it up if needed).

2 Add the water and miso paste to the pan and simmer. Add the chicken and cook for 4 minutes. Add the sweetcorn, pak choi, eggs noodles & peas and simmer for 4-5 minutes or until the chicken is cooked through and the noodles & vegetables are tender.

3 Check the seasoning, spoon into bowls and serve with lime wedges.

CHEFS NOTE
You could use cooked chicken for this soup. Just shred it and add to the pan when you add the vegetables & noodles.

SMOKED SAUSAGE & SOUP

220 calories per serving

Ingredients

- 200g/7oz low fat smoked pork sausages
- 1 onion, sliced
- 125g/4oz carrots, peeled & diced
- 1 garlic clove, crushed
- 400g/14oz tinned lentils, drained & rinsed
- ½ tsp crushed chilli flakes
- 1.25lt/5 cups vegetable or chicken stock
- Low cal cooking oil spray
- Salt & pepper to taste

Method

1 Preheat the grill to a medium heat and cook the sausages for 8-10 minutes or until cooked through. When they are ready, slice into thin discs and put to one side.

2 In the meantime using a little low cal spray, gently sauté the onion, carrots & garlic in a large non-stick saucepan for a few minutes until softened (add a splash of water to loosen it up if needed).

3 Sauté for a few minutes before adding the lentils, chilli & stock and cook for 5 minutes.

4 Tip the soup into a blender or food processor and whizz until you have a completely smooth texture.

5 Return the soup to the pan along with the sliced sausages. Simmer for 5 minutes or until everything is piping hot and cooked through.

6 Add a little more stock if needed, check the seasoning and serve.

CHEFS NOTE

Some smoked sausage comes vacuum packed ready to steam rather than grill. Follow the cooking instructions on the packet.

TRADITIONAL MULLIGATAWNY SOUP

205 calories per serving

Ingredients

- 1 onion, sliced
- 2 garlic cloves, crushed
- 2 stalks of celery, chopped
- 200g/7oz carrots, peeled & chopped
- 200g/7oz turnip, peeled & chopped
- 200g/7oz sweet potatoes, peeled & chopped
- 1 tbsp medium curry powder

- 1 tbsp tomato puree
- 50g/2oz rice
- 1 eating apple, peeled & cored
- 1lt/4 cups vegetable or chicken stock
- 4 tbsp fat free Greek yogurt
- Low cal cooking oil spray
- Salt & pepper to taste

Method

1 Using a little low cal spray gently sauté the onions, garlic & celery in a large non-stick saucepan for a few minutes until softened.

2 Add all the other ingredients, except the Greek yogurt, and simmer for 12-16 minutes or until the rice is tender.

3 Tip the soup into a blender or food processor and whizz until you have a completely smooth texture.

4 Check the seasoning and serve with a tablespoon of Greek yogurt swirled though the soup.

CHEFS NOTE

Try serving with a dollop of mango chutney too.

LENTIL & BABY SPINACH SOUP

215 calories per serving

Ingredients

- 1 tbsp low fat 'butter' spread
- 1 onion, sliced
- 1 garlic clove, crushed
- 200g/7oz puy lentils
- ½ tsp crushed sea salt
- 1lt/4 cups vegetable or chicken stock
- 200g/7oz baby spinach leaves
- 2 tbsp freshly chopped basil
- Salt & pepper to taste

Method

1 Gently heat the 'butter' in a large non-stick saucepan and add the onions & garlic. Sauté for a few minutes before adding the puy lentils, salt & stock.

2 Simmer for 15-20 minutes, add the spinach and continue to cook for a few minutes or until the lentils are tender and the spinach is cooked through.

3 Tip the soup into a blender or food processor and whizz until you have a completely smooth texture.

4 Add a little more stock if needed, check the seasoning and serve with basil sprinkled over the top.

CHEFS NOTE
Swirl through a little low fat cream for an extra creamy finish.

BEST CRAB & SWEETCORN SOUP

265 calories per serving

Ingredients

- 1 tbsp low fat 'butter' spread
- 4 shallots, chopped
- 1 garlic clove, crushed
- 1 tsp mild curry powder
- 200g/7oz potatoes, peeled & diced

- 300g/11oz sweetcorn
- 750ml/3 cups vegetable or chicken stock
- 250ml/1 cup low fat cream
- 150g/5oz tinned crabmeat, drained
- Salt & pepper to taste

Method

1 Gently heat the olive oil in a large non-stick saucepan and sauté the shallots and garlic for a few minutes until softened.

2 Stir through the curry powder, add the potatoes, sweetcorn & stock and simmer for 10-12 minutes or until the potatoes are tender.

3 Tip the soup into a blender or food processor and whizz until you have a completely smooth texture.

4 Return the soup to the pan and on a very gently heat stir through the cream.

5 Check the seasoning and serve with the crab meat flaked over the top of each bowl.

CHEFS NOTE
Use the best crabmeat you can find. Tinned is fine but fresh is even better!

CURRIED, HONEY PARSNIP SOUP

205 calories per serving

Ingredients

- 1 tbsp olive oil
- 1 onion, sliced
- 1 garlic clove, crushed
- 1 tbsp mild curry powder
- 500g/1lb 2oz parsnips, peeled & diced
- 200g/7oz potatoes, peeled & diced
- 1 tbsp honey
- 1lt/4 cups vegetable or chicken stock
- 2 tbsp fat free crème fraiche
- Salt & pepper to taste

Method

1 Gently heat the olive oil in a large non-stick saucepan and sauté the onions & garlic for a few minutes until softened.

2 Stir through the curry powder, add the parsnips, potatoes, honey & stock and simmer for 10-12 minutes or until the parsnips are tender.

3 Tip the soup into a blender or food processor along with the crème fraiche and whizz until you have a completely smooth texture.

4 Check the seasoning and serve.

CHEFS NOTE
Use medium or hot curry powder if you prefer.

COCONUT MILK & SHRIMP SOUP

280 calories per serving

Ingredients

- 1 tbsp olive oil
- 1 garlic clove, crushed
- ½ tsp crushed chilli flakes
- 300g/11oz peeled prawns, roughly chopped
- ½ tsp crushed sea salt
- 4 spring onions/scallions, finely chopped
- 500ml/2 cups vegetable or chicken stock
- 500ml/2 cups low fat coconut milk
- Zest of 1 lime
- Salt & pepper to taste

Method

1 Gently heat the oil in a large non-stick saucepan and add the garlic, chilli flakes, prawns, salt & spring onions.

2 Sauté for a couple of minutes before adding the stock & coconut milk. Cover and leave on a very low heat to cook for 5- 6 minutes or until the prawns are cooked through.

3 Check the seasoning and serve with the lime zest sprinkled over the top.

CHEFS NOTE

Add a little more stock if you want the soup to go further.

CHUNKY MINESTRONE

250 calories per serving

Ingredients

- 2 onions, sliced
- 3 garlic cloves, crushed
- 75g/3oz lean, back bacon, finely chopped
- 1 tsp dried mixed herbs
- 300g/11oz potatoes, peeled & diced
- 300g/11oz carrots, peeled & diced
- 4 celery stalks, chopped

- 2 tbsp tomato puree/paste
- 400g/1oz tinned chopped tomatoes
- 1lt/4 cups vegetable or chicken stock
- 75g/3oz soup pasta
- Low cal cooking oil spray
- Salt & pepper to taste

Method

1 Using a little low cal spray gently sauté the onion, garlic, bacon, herbs, potatoes, carrots & celery in a large non-stick saucepan for a few minutes until the onions soften and the bacon is cooked (add a splash of water to the pan if you need to loosen it up).

2 Stir through the tomato puree, add the chopped tomatoes, stock & pasta and simmer for 15-20minutes or until everything is cooked through and tender.

3 Check the seasoning and serve.

CHEFS NOTE

Use any mix of vegetables you prefer for this rustic soup...also good served with some grated Parmesan cheese!

SWEET POTATO & CHORIZO SOUP

205 calories per serving

Ingredients

- 2 celery stalks, chopped
- 1 leek, chopped
- 75g/3oz chorizo, chopped
- 200g/7oz carrots peeled & dice
- 800g/1¾lb sweet potatoes, peeled & diced
- 2 tbsp balsamic vinegar
- 1 tsp each paprika & cumin
- 400g/14oz tinned chopped tomatoes
- 2 tbsp tomato puree/paste
- 1lt/4 cups vegetable or chicken stock
- Low cal cooking oil spray
- Salt & pepper to taste

Method

1 Gently sauté the celery, leek, chorizo, carrots & sweet potatoes in a large non-stick saucepan, with a little low cal spray, for a few minutes until the onions soften (add a splash of water to the pan if you need to loosen it up).

2 Stir through the balsamic vinegar, ground spices, chopped tomatoes, tomato puree & stock and simmer for 15-20 minutes or until the sweet potatoes are cooked through.

3 Check the seasoning and serve.

CHEFS NOTE
Add a pinch salt and brown sugar to balance the acidity of the tomatoes if needed.

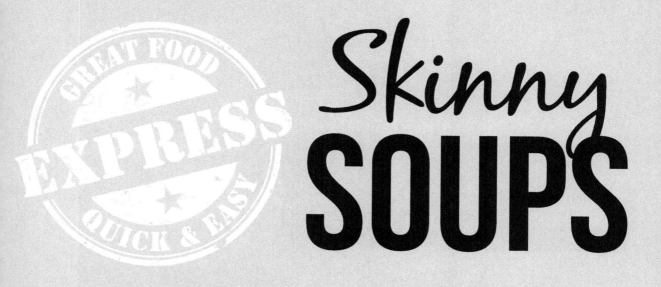

Skinny SOUPS

GREAT FOOD
EXPRESS
QUICK & EASY

UNDER 400 CALORIES

SEAFOOD CHOWDER

325 calories per serving

Ingredients

- 1 onion, sliced
- 75g/3oz lean, back bacon, finely chopped
- 2 onions, sliced
- 250g/9oz potatoes, peeled & chopped
- 150g/5oz sweetcorn
- ½ tsp each paprika, cayenne pepper & dried thyme
- 750ml/3 cups, vegetable or chicken stock

- 400g/14oz mixed seafood
- 500ml/2 cups semi skimmed/half fat milk
- 2 tbsp fat free crème fraiche
- 4 tbsp freshly chopped chives
- Low cal cooking oil spray
- Salt & pepper to taste

Method

1 Using a little low cal spray gently sauté the onions & bacon in a large non-stick saucepan for a few minutes until the onions soften and the bacon is cooked.

2 Add the potatoes, sweetcorn, herbs, spices & stock and simmer 10 minutes.

3 Use the back of a large spoon or fork to crush some of the potatoes and combine well.

4 Add the seafood & milk and gently simmer for 3-4 minutes or until the seafood is cooked through and the vegetables are tender.

5 Stir through the crème fraiche and chives. Check the seasoning and serve.

CHEFS NOTE
Bags of fresh or frozen mixed seafood are readily available in most stores.

TOFU LAKSA

340 calories per serving

Ingredients

- 2 bunches spring onions/scallions
- 2 garlic cloves
- 2 lemongrass stalks, trimmed
- 1 tbsp tomato puree/paste
- 1 tsp ground coriander/cilantro
- 1 tbsp tamarind paste
- 300g/11oz fresh tomatoes
- 1 red chilli, deseeded

- 500ml/2 cups vegetable or chicken stock
- 500ml/2 cups low fat coconut milk
- 1 tbsp Thai fish sauce
- 2 tbsp soy sauce
- 125g/5oz tofu, cubed
- 200g/7oz thin egg noodles
- Salt & pepper to taste

Method

1 Place the spring onions, garlic cloves, lemon grass stalks, tomato puree, coriander, tamarind paste, fresh tomatoes & chilli in a food processor and pulse until finely chopped into a fresh paste.

2 Using a little low cal spray gently sauté the paste in a large non-stick saucepan for 5 minutes.

3 Add the rest of the ingredients and simmer for 3-5 minutes or until everything is cooked through and piping hot.

4 Check the seasoning and serve.

CHEFS NOTE
Try serving with some freshly chopped chilli or lime wedges.

EASY EGG RAMEN

325 calories per serving

Ingredients

- 4 free range eggs
- 2 garlic cloves, crushed
- 2 red chillies, deseeded & finely chopped
- ½ tsp ground ginger
- 4 tbsp miso paste
- 1.25lt/5 cups boiling water
- 125g/4oz oyster mushrooms, finely sliced

- 1 bunch spring onions/scallions, finely sliced
- 200g/7oz thick udon noodles
- 4 tbsp freshly chopped chives
- 200g/7oz fresh beansprouts
- Salt & pepper to taste

Method

1 Put the eggs into a pan of water and cook until hardboiled.

2 Meanwhile add the boiling water and miso paste to a non-stick saucepan and stir well on a medium heat.

3 Add all the ingredients, except the eggs & beansprouts, to the pan and cook for 3-4 minutes or until everything is cooked through and piping hot.

4 Peel the boiled eggs and cut in half lengthways. Add the beansprouts to the pan and cook for a minute longer.

5 Check the seasoning, spoon into bowls and serve with 2 boiled egg halves sitting on top of each portion.

CHEFS NOTE
Break the noodles into pieces to make the ramen easier to eat!

BURNS NIGHT BROTH

310
calories per
serving

Ingredients

- 1 tbsp olive oil
- ½ onion, sliced
- 200g/7oz potatoes, peeled & finely diced
- 200g/7oz carrots, peeled & finely diced
- 200g/7oz swede peeled & finely diced
- 1lt/4 cups vegetable or chicken stock
- 300g/11oz haggis
- 4 tsp freshly chopped flat leaf parsley
- Salt & pepper to taste

Method

1 Gently heat the olive oil in a large non-stick saucepan and sauté the vegetables for a few minutes until softened.

2 Add the stock and simmer for 5 minutes. Add the haggis and cook for a further 10 minutes or until everything is tender and cooked through.

3 Check the seasoning, divide into bowls and serve with the chopped parsley sprinkled over the top.

CHEFS NOTE
Perfect for a January Burn's night celebration.

HONEY BEEF UDON SOUP

390 calories per serving

Ingredients

- ½ tsp ground ginger
- 1.25lt/5 cups vegetable or chicken stock
- 150g/5oz peas
- 4 tbsp soy sauce
- 1 tsp olive oil

- 3 tbsp honey
- 300g/11oz sirloin steak
- 200g/7oz thick udon noodles
- Salt & pepper to taste

Method

1 Add the ginger, stock, peas & soy sauce to a saucepan and simmer over a gentle heat.

2 Meanwhile place a non-stick saucepan on a high heat until it is smoking hot. Brush the steak with the olive oil and season well.

3 Add the steak in the pan and cook for 2 minutes each side. Place the cooked steak on a chopping board to rest and brush with honey.

4 Add the noodles and simmer for 2 minutes. Meanwhile use a sharp knife to slice the steak very thinly.

5 Divide the soup into bowls and lay the steak over the top. Serve immediately.

CHEFS NOTE
Alter the cooking time of the steak to suit your own taste.

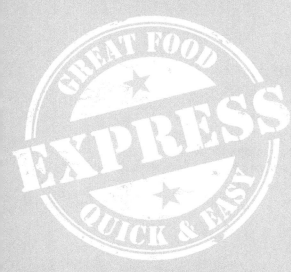

Skinny SOUP

STOCK

It's not necessary to make your own stock to create good soup, quality shop-bought stock works well too. However if you do want to have a go at making homemade stock here are some basic recipes.

BASIC VEGETABLE STOCK

Ingredients

- 1 tbsp olive oil
- 1 onion, chopped
- 1 leek, chopped
- 1 carrot, chopped
- 1 small bulb fennel, chopped
- 3 garlic cloves, crushed
- 1 tbsp black peppercorns

- 75g/3oz mushrooms
- 2 sticks celery, chopped
- 3 tomatoes, diced
- 2 tbsp freshly chopped flat leaf parsley
- 2 bay leaves
- 3lt/12 cups water

Method

Gently sauté the onions, leeks, carrots and fennel in the olive oil for a few minutes in a large lidded saucepan. Add all the other ingredients, cover and bring to the boil. Leave to gently simmer for 20 minutes with the lid on. Cool for a little while. Pour the contents through a sieve and store the finished stock liquid in the fridge for a couple of days or freeze in batches.

BASIC CHICKEN STOCK

- 1 tbsp olive oil
- 1 left over roast chicken carcass
- 2 carrots, chopped
- 2 onions, halved
- 2 stalks celery, chopped

- 10 black peppercorns
- 2 bay leaves
- 2 tbsp freshly chopped parsley
- 1 tsp freshly chopped thyme
- 3lt/12 cups water

Method

Gently sauté the onions, carrots and celery in the olive oil for a few minutes in a large lidded saucepan. Break the chicken carcass up into pieces and add to the pan along with all the other ingredients, cover and bring to the boil. Leave to very gently simmer for 1hr with the lid on. Cool for a little while. Pour the contents through a sieve and store the finished stock liquid in the fridge for a couple of days or freeze in batches. You may find you need to skim a little fat from the top of the stock after cooking.

BASIC FISH STOCK

Ingredients

- 1 tbsp olive oil
- 450g/1lb fish bones, heads carcasses etc (avoid oily fish when making stock)
- 4 leeks, chopped
- 1 fennel bulb, chopped
- 4 carrots, chopped
- 2 tbsp freshly chopped parsley
- 250ml/1 cup dry white wine
- 2.5lt/10 cups water

Method

Gently sauté the carrots, leeks and fennel in the olive oil for a few minutes in a large lidded saucepan. Clean the fish bones to ensure there is no blood as this can 'spoil' the stock. Add all the other ingredients, cover and bring to the boil. Leave to very gently simmer for 1hr with the lid on. Cool for a little while. Pour the contents through a sieve and store the finished stock liquid in the fridge for a couple of days or freeze in batches. You may find you need to skim a little fat from the top of the stock after cooking.

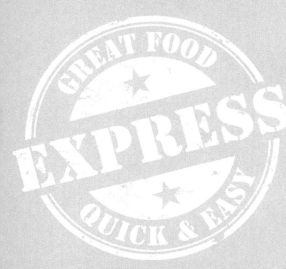

Skinny SOUPS

GARNISH

HOMEMADE CROUTONS

50 calories per portion

Ingredients

- 4 slices thick wholemeal bread
- 2 tsp garlic powder
- 2 tsp dried mixed herbs
- 1 tsp crushed sea salt flakes
- Low cal cooking oil spray

Method

1 Preheat the oven to 350f/180c/Gas 4

2 Remove the crusts with a knife and cube the bread into crouton-sized pieces.

3 Spray the bread cubes with some low cal oil and place in a plastic bag with the garlic powder, herbs and salt. Give the bag a good shake until all the bread is covered with the seasoning.

4 Lay the bread cubes out on a non-stick baking tray and cook in the preheated oven for 13-15 minutes or until the croutons are crisp and golden brown.

5 Allow to cool. Use straightway or store in an airtight container for up to 3 days.

CHEFS NOTE

You could add some grated Parmesan to the seasoning for extra taste.

CORIANDER GREMOLATA

35
calories per portion

Ingredients

- 4 tbsp lemon zest
- 3 tbsp freshly chopped coriander/cilantro
- 4 garlic cloves, crushed
- 2 tbsp extra virgin olive oil
- ½ tsp crushed sea salt flakes

Method

1 Mix everything together until really well combined. Try using a small clean lidded jar and shaking.

2 Add a little more oil if needed and feel free to alter the balance of salt, garlic and lemon to suit your own taste.

CHEFS NOTE

This is great sprinkled or stirred through soup just prior to serving.

HONEY FRIED ONIONS

40
calories per portion

Ingredients

- 1 tbsp olive oil
- 2 mild white onions, sliced
- 1 tbsp honey
- 2 tbsp balsamic vinegar

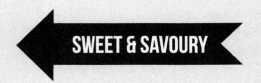

SWEET & SAVOURY

Method

1 Heat the olive oil in a non-stick frying pan and gently sauté for 10-15 minutes until softened and browned.

2 Stir through the honey and balsamic vinegar. Increase the heat and cook for 2 minutes longer.

3 Remove from the pan and store in the fridge for up to three days.

CHEFS NOTE

Fry the onions quite hard after you add the honey to brown them up ready to garnish. Either serve warm or allow to cool and serve straight from the fridge.

ROASTED CHICKPEAS

40
calories per portion

Ingredients

- 200g/7oz tinned chickpeas, drained
- 1-2 tsp crushed sea salt flakes
- 1 tbsp olive oil
- Low cal cooking oil spray

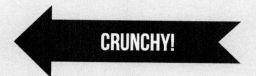

CRUNCHY!

Method

1 Preheat the oven to 350f/180c/Gas 4

2 Dry off the chickpeas and combine with the sea salt and olive oil.

3 Spread out on a baking tray, place into the oven and cook for 25-30 minutes or until they turn brown & crisp.

4 Use straight away or store in an airtight container for up to 3 days.

CHEFS NOTE
Keep an eye on the chickpeas when they are in the oven and turn a few times to prevent burning.

CONVERSION CHART: DRY INGREDIENTS

Metric	Imperial
7g	¼ oz
15g	½ oz
20g	¾ oz
25g	1 oz
40g	1½oz
50g	2oz
60g	2½oz
75g	3oz
100g	3½oz
125g	4oz
140g	4½oz
150g	5oz
165g	5½oz
175g	6oz
200g	7oz
225g	8oz
250g	9oz
275g	10oz
300g	11oz
350g	12oz
375g	13oz
400g	14oz

Metric	Imperial
425g	15oz
450g	1lb
500g	1lb 2oz
550g	1¼lb
600g	1lb 5oz
650g	1lb 7oz
675g	1½lb
700g	1lb 9oz
750g	1lb 11oz
800g	1¾lb
900g	2lb
1kg	2¼lb
1.1kg	2½lb
1.25kg	2¾lb
1.35kg	3lb
1.5kg	3lb 6oz
1.8kg	4lb
2kg	4½lb
2.25kg	5lb
2.5kg	5½lb
2.75kg	6lb

CONVERSION CHART: LIQUID MEASURES

Metric	Imperial	US
25ml	1fl oz	
60ml	2fl oz	¼ cup
75ml	2½ fl oz	
100ml	3½fl oz	
120ml	4fl oz	½ cup
150ml	5fl oz	
175ml	6fl oz	
200ml	7fl oz	
250ml	8½ fl oz	1 cup
300ml	10½ fl oz	
360ml	12½ fl oz	
400ml	14fl oz	
450ml	15½ fl oz	
600ml	1 pint	
750ml	1¼ pint	3 cups
1 litre	1½ pints	4 cups

Other COOKNATION TITLES

If you enjoyed 'The Skinny Express Soup Recipe Book' we'd really appreciate your feedback. Reviews help others decide if this is the right book for them so a moment of your time would be appreciated.

Thank you.

You may also be interested in other 'Skinny' titles in the CookNation series. You can find all the following great titles by searching under 'CookNation'.

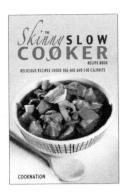

THE SKINNY SLOW COOKER RECIPE BOOK

Delicious Recipes Under 300, 400 And 500 Calories.

Paperback / eBook

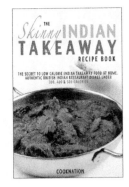

THE SKINNY INDIAN TAKEAWAY RECIPE BOOK

Authentic British Indian Restaurant Dishes Under 300, 400 And 500 Calories. The Secret To Low Calorie Indian Takeaway Food At Home.

Paperback / eBook

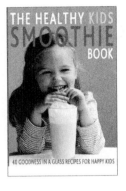

THE HEALTHY KIDS SMOOTHIE BOOK

40 Delicious Goodness In A Glass Recipes for Happy Kids.

eBook

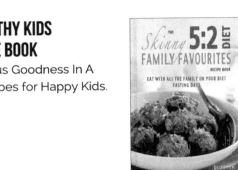
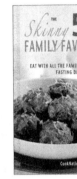

THE SKINNY 5:2 FAST DIET FAMILY FAVOURITES RECIPE BOOK

Eat With All The Family On Your Diet Fasting Days.

Paperback / eBook

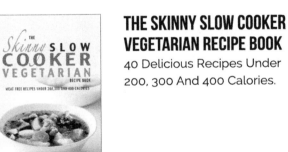

THE SKINNY SLOW COOKER VEGETARIAN RECIPE BOOK

40 Delicious Recipes Under 200, 300 And 400 Calories.

Paperback / eBook

THE PALEO DIET FOR BEGINNERS SLOW COOKER RECIPE BOOK

Gluten Free, Everyday Essential Slow Cooker Paleo Recipes For Beginners.

eBook

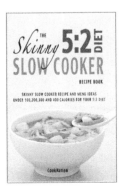

THE SKINNY 5:2 SLOW COOKER RECIPE BOOK

Skinny Slow Cooker Recipe And Menu Ideas Under 100, 200, 300 & 400 Calories For Your 5:2 Diet.

Paperback / eBook

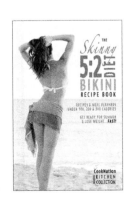

THE SKINNY 5:2 BIKINI DIET RECIPE BOOK

Recipes & Meal Planners Under 100, 200 & 300 Calories. Get Ready For Summer & Lose Weight...FAST!

Paperback / eBook

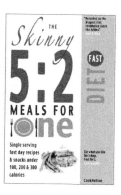

THE SKINNY 5:2 FAST DIET MEALS FOR ONE

Single Serving Fast Day Recipes & Snacks Under 100, 200 & 300 Calories.

Paperback / eBook

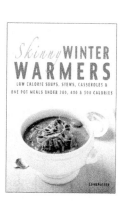

THE SKINNY HALOGEN OVEN FAMILY FAVOURITES RECIPE BOOK

Healthy, Low Calorie Family Meal-Time Halogen Oven Recipes Under 300, 400 and 500 Calories.

Paperback / eBook

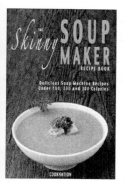

THE SKINNY 5:2 FAST DIET VEGETARIAN MEALS FOR ONE

Single Serving Fast Day Recipes & Snacks Under 100, 200 & 300 Calories.

Paperback / eBook

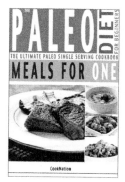

THE PALEO DIET FOR BEGINNERS MEALS FOR ONE

The Ultimate Paleo Single Serving Cookbook.

Paperback / eBook

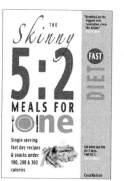

THE SKINNY SOUP MAKER RECIPE BOOK

Delicious Low Calorie, Healthy and Simple Soup Recipes Under 100, 200 and 300 Calories. Perfect For Any Diet and Weight Loss Plan.

Paperback / eBook

THE PALEO DIET FOR BEGINNERS HOLIDAYS

Thanksgiving, Christmas & New Year Paleo Friendly Recipes.
eBook

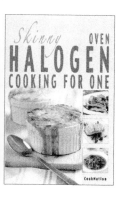

SKINNY HALOGEN OVEN COOKING FOR ONE

Single Serving, Healthy, Low Calorie Halogen Oven RecipesUnder 200, 300 and 400 Calories.

Paperback / eBook

SKINNY WINTER WARMERS RECIPE BOOK

Soups, Stews, Casseroles & One Pot Meals Under 300, 400 & 500 Calories.

Paperback / eBook

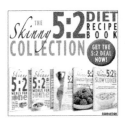

THE SKINNY 5:2 DIET RECIPE BOOK COLLECTION

All The 5:2 Fast Diet Recipes You'll Ever Need. All Under 100, 200, 300, 400 And 500 Calories.
eBook

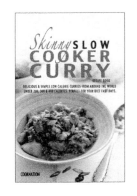

THE SKINNY SLOW COOKER CURRY RECIPE BOOK

Low Calorie Curries From Around The World.

Paperback / eBook

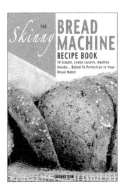

THE SKINNY BREAD MACHINE RECIPE BOOK

70 Simple, Lower Calorie, Healthy Breads...Baked To Perfection In Your Bread Maker.

Paperback / eBook

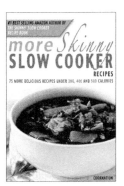

MORE SKINNY SLOW COOKER RECIPES

75 More Delicious Recipes Under 300, 400 & 500 Calories.

Paperback / eBook

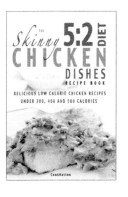

THE SKINNY 5:2 DIET CHICKEN DISHES RECIPE BOOK

Delicious Low Calorie Chicken Dishes Under 300, 400 & 500 Calories.

Paperback / eBook

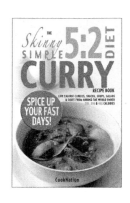

THE SKINNY 5:2 CURRY RECIPE BOOK

Spice Up Your Fast Days With Simple Low Calorie Curries, Snacks, Soups, Salads & Sides Under 200, 300 & 400 Calories.

Paperback / eBook

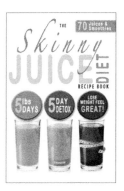

THE SKINNY JUICE DIET RECIPE BOOK

5lbs, 5 Days. The Ultimate Kick- Start Diet and Detox Plan to Lose Weight & Feel Great!

Paperback / eBook

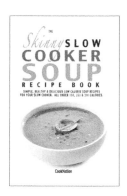

THE SKINNY SLOW COOKER SOUP RECIPE BOOK

Simple, Healthy & Delicious Low Calorie Soup Recipes For Your Slow Cooker. All Under 100, 200 & 300 Calories.

Paperback / eBook

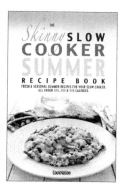

THE SKINNY SLOW COOKER SUMMER RECIPE BOOK

Fresh & Seasonal Summer Recipes For Your Slow Cooker. All Under 300, 400 And 500 Calories.

Paperback / eBook

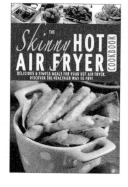

THE SKINNY HOT AIR FRYER COOKBOOK

Delicious & Simple Meals For Your Hot Air Fryer: Discover The Healthier Way To Fry.

Paperback / eBook

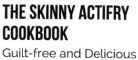

THE SKINNY ACTIFRY COOKBOOK

Guilt-free and Delicious ActiFry Recipe Ideas: Discover The Healthier Way to Fry!

Paperback / eBook

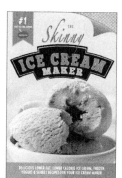

THE SKINNY ICE CREAM MAKER

Delicious Lower Fat, Lower Calorie Ice Cream, Frozen Yogurt & Sorbet Recipes For Your Ice Cream Maker.

Paperback / eBook

THE SKINNY 15 MINUTE MEALS RECIPE BOOK

Delicious, Nutritious & Super-Fast Meals in 15 Minutes Or Less. All Under 300, 400 & 500 Calories.

Paperback / eBook

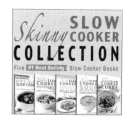

THE SKINNY SLOW COOKER COLLECTION

5 Fantastic Books of Delicious, Diet-friendly Skinny Slow Cooker Recipes: ALL Under 200, 300, 400 & 500 Calories!
eBook

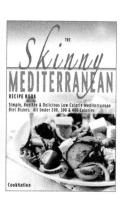

THE SKINNY MEDITERRANEAN RECIPE BOOK

Simple, Healthy & Delicious Low Calorie Mediterranean Diet Dishes. All Under 200, 300 & 400 Calories.

Paperback / eBook

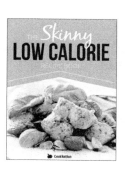

THE SKINNY LOW CALORIE RECIPE BOOK

Great Tasting, Simple & Healthy Meals Under 300, 400 & 500 Calories. Perfect For Any Calorie Controlled Diet.

Paperback / eBook

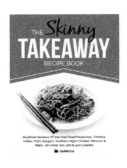

THE SKINNY TAKEAWAY RECIPE BOOK

Healthier Versions Of Your Fast Food Favourites: All Under 300, 400 & 500 Calories.

Paperback / eBook

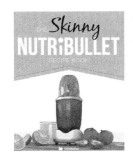

THE SKINNY NUTRIBULLET RECIPE BOOK

80+ Delicious & Nutritious Healthy Smoothie Recipes. Burn Fat, Lose Weight and Feel Great!

Paperback / eBook

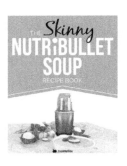

THE SKINNY NUTRIBULLET SOUP RECIPE BOOK

Delicious, Quick & Easy, Single Serving Soups & Pasta Sauces For Your Nutribullet. All Under 100, 200, 300 & 400 Calories!

Paperback / eBook

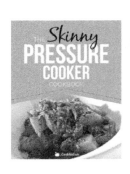

THE SKINNY PRESSURE COOKER COOKBOOK

USA ONLY

Low Calorie, Healthy & Delicious Meals, Sides & Desserts. All Under 300, 400 & 500 Calories.

Paperback / eBook

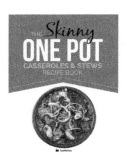

THE SKINNY ONE-POT RECIPE BOOK

Simple & Delicious, One-Pot Meals. All Under 300, 400 & 500 Calories

Paperback / eBook

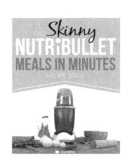

THE SKINNY NUTRIBULLET MEALS IN MINUTES RECIPE BOOK

Quick & Easy, Single Serving Suppers, Snacks, Sauces, Salad Dressings & More Using Your Nutribullet. All Under 300, 400 & 500 Calories

Paperback / eBook

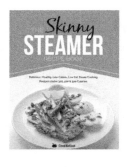

THE SKINNY STEAMER RECIPE BOOK

Healthy, Low Calorie, Low Fat Steam Cooking Recipes Under 300, 400 & 500 Calories.

Paperback / eBook

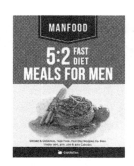

MANFOOD: 5:2 FAST DIET MEALS FOR MEN

Simple & Delicious, Fuss Free, Fast Day Recipes For Men Under 200, 300, 400 & 500 Calories.

Paperback / eBook

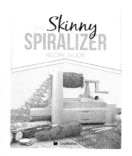

THE SKINNY SPIRALIZER RECIPE BOOK

Delicious Spiralizer Inspired Low Calorie Recipes For One. All Under 200, 300, 400 & 500 Calories

Paperback / eBook

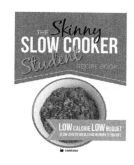

THE SKINNY SLOW COOKER STUDENT RECIPE BOOK

Delicious, Simple, Low Calorie, Low Budget, Slow Cooker Meals For Hungry Students. All Under 300, 400 & 500 Calories

Paperback / eBook

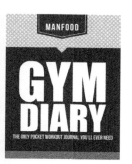

MANFOOD: GYM DIARY:

The Only Pocket Workout Journal You'll Ever Need

Paperback / eBook

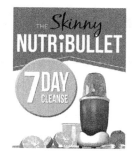

THE SKINNY NUTRIBULLET 7 DAY CLEANSE

Calorie Counted Cleanse & Detox Plan: Smoothies, Soups & Meals to Lose Weight & Feel Great Fast. Real Food. Real Results

Paperback / eBook

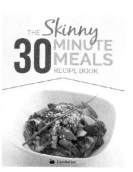

THE SKINNY 30 MINUTE MEALS RECIPE BOOK

Great Food, Easy Recipes, Prepared & Cooked In 30 Minutes Or Less. All Under 300, 400 & 500 Calories

Paperback / eBook

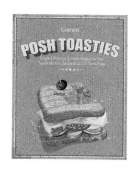

POSH TOASTIES

Simple & Delicious Gourmet Recipes For Your Toastie Machine, Sandwich Grill Or Panini Press

Paperback / eBook

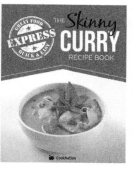

THE SKINNY EXPRESS CURRY RECIPE BOOK

Quick & Easy Authentic Low Fat Indian Dishes Under 300, 400 & 500 Calories

Paperback / eBook

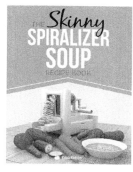

THE SKINNY SPIRALIZER SOUP RECIPE BOOK

Delicious Spiralizer Inspired Soup Recipes All Under 100, 200, 300 & 400 Calories

Paperback / eBook

Printed in Great Britain
by Amazon